I0788312

Table of Contents

Introduction

When you make the decision to hire a personal trainer, it can be a little overwhelming. You're trusting them to give your current lifestyle a complete overhaul and help to transform you into a stronger, healthier person.

It's okay to be nervous when taking such a big and important step. Before you do though, you're going to want to have a good idea of what you can expect.

It's not easy to ask someone else to help you change for the better. After all, as humans, we tend to be creatures of habit. But sometimes, it's important to step back and take a closer look at those habits, acknowledging the fact that they aren't always as good as they could be.

Recognizing your faults, and creating that motivation for change is why having a personal trainer can be instrumental in your success.

Personal trainers are on the outside looking in, and with their knowledge and skillset, they can tweak the small things you may not notice, to make a greater impact then you could ever imagine. Keep in mind that they are health professionals and their advice is usually based on scientific research and proven theories.

This report is not only for those of you who need to know what to expect from a good, experienced personal trainer, but it is also for the people out there just beginning to dip their toes into the idea of self-improvement and better fitness and nutritional habits.

Let's take an inside look into some of the tips and tricks that personal trainers share with their clients!

Important Note: It's important that you seek the advice and approval from your health care provider prior to making any drastic changes to your diet or exercise.

Tip #1: Visualize Your Goal

You don't want to just state your goal; you want to truly see it materializing right in front of you.

It's a good idea to take some time and write down what you want out of your relationship with a personal trainer as well as what health goals you are striving for.

It's even better when you revisit those goals again and again to remind yourself of the healthy new you that you are striving to be. It does you no good to jot these goals down and then stow them away.

Out of sight, out of mind.

Vision boards have been popping up all over the internet. These boards are places to visualize the goals that people have, to keep them focused along the way. Well, those boards aren't just for people who have a bucket list full of travel destinations. They're also for people who have health and nutrition goals as well!

One of the things that personal trainers tell their clients to practice, is visualization. Take the written or verbal goals that you have, and bring them to life through visual aids.

For example, if a client wants to lose 50 pounds, then they may suggest the following: get a large poster board, print off five pictures of 10-pound bags of rice or flour, and glue them to the board.

Whenever they look at it, not only will they be reminded of their long-term goal, but they'll also be able to physically see how much ten pounds of weight loss really is.

Perhaps the personal trainer's client wants to look like she did in high school. In this case, they might have them hang up a picture of their younger days where they're most likely to see it on a regular basis. In addition to that, a personal trainer may suggest that they include pictures of workouts that will help them achieve this goal.

What is your main goal?

Health goal specifics vary from person to person, but in general, the main goal whether weight loss, weight gain, or better eating habits, it is always to become a healthier version of you.

Hiring a personal trainer doesn't necessarily mean that you want to lose weight. Personal trainers deal with weight gain, muscle gain, heart health, and many other areas.

When you're deciding on your goals and what you want to pass over to the trainer, ask yourself the following questions.

- **What is my ideal weight?** Schedule an appointment with your physician and discuss with them what your personal, ideal Body Mass Index and Weight should be. While you can easily search the internet to find out what your weight should be, your healthcare professional can look at your medical history and take everything into consideration before giving you a number. This is especially important if you're on medication that slows down your metabolism. Once you have that number, write it into your Vision Board.

- **What areas of my body need the most work?** If you want slender arms and legs, then print out stock images of your ideal look and post them on your Vision Board. The same goes for any other body part that you want to change. Remember, be realistic with your expectations and base them on your body, not the model in the picture.

- **Do I want to train for a specific sport?** If you're meeting with a personal trainer because you want to participate in a specific sport, then print a picture of that sport out and post it on your Vision Board. For example, if you want to run a marathon, then post a picture of marathon runners on your board. Fliers for a specific marathon you wish to participate in are also good motivators. But you should know there is a difference between personal trainers and sport specific trainers.

Remember, seeing is believing, and believing drives you to work that much harder to achieve your goals. So, whatever your goal is, make your Vision Board and hang it proudly where you can see it every day.

Tip #2: Reprogram Your Mind

Our bodies are designed to protect us, and our brains are our strongest armor. The brain automatically attempts to shield us from anything that creates a feeling of anxiety and nervousness.

Changes to our normal way of life and routine can create those exact feelings. When your brain senses that, it will attempt to derail you from those changes as protection for the unknown.

But don't let it.

When you meet with your personal trainer, discuss the issues of change. Repetition and a positive mindset can help settle those anxious feelings. It's important for you to develop your own positive routine in order to reprogram your mind to understand you are doing what's best for it. Whether it's having to wake up earlier for an exercise session, or not indulging in a quick trip to the fast food restaurant, your personal trainer will be there to help you break the negative cycle with minimal anxiety.

A personal trainer will help you tackle the hardest parts of sticking to a healthy lifestyle.

Recognize What Holds You Back: If work often gets in the way of exercising, the trainer may have you commit to a specific time, every day, to exercise. This will take out the interference of work, and open you up to a new routine.

Retrain Your Way of Thinking: Whenever you're not in the mood to workout, a personal trainer will motivate you through a dedication not just to them, but to yourself as well. As soon as your brain begins to bargain with your workout, get moving.

A body in motion, stays in motion. Your trainer may have you create a list of affirmations you can repeat to yourself, when you are feeling particularly lazy or unmotivated. This is only natural, and will lesson over time.

Tear Up Your List of Excuses: Personal trainers oftentimes have you participate in a symbolic gesture for your brain to connect to that negativity and assist in helping you continue your path.

By writing down all the reasons you have to NOT workout, and then tearing those up, you are symbolizing your intent to bypass that reasoning and do what you know is best for your body.

Nobody is perfect, and it's only normal to have days where working out seems like torture. But a good personal trainer will not only acknowledge this, but will go out of their way to help you overcome those feelings!

Tip #3: Take Baby Steps

The decision to turn your life around is exciting, but can also be overwhelming. Deciding to change your health and eating habits is a big step and can often be decided on in just a moment's notice. But once you've decided what you want, start to slow down the process just a bit.

Here are a few ways to start out slow.

Replace One Meal a Day: Do you get a muffin with your coffee-to-go order every day? Consider having a bowl of oatmeal and some form of protein on the side before hitting up that drive-thru. You'll be too full to order a muffin, but you can still enjoy your coffee.

Start Your Day with A 5-Minute Cardio Session: If you are new to exercising and really need to take it slow, then consider doing a five-minute cardio burn every morning. There are plenty of options readily available online, and doing so will help prepare you for your longer, more intense sessions with your personal trainer.

Drink More Water: You have probably heard this hundreds of times, but getting enough water really is one of the most important things you can do for yourself every day.

It's not an easy switch from soda, though. Start out slow by replacing an eight-ounce cup of water for one serving of soda per day. From there, move up as quickly as you can, until water is your main source of hydration.

Tip #4: Communication is Key

It's not easy asking for help, but that's what personal trainers are supposed to do, help you. Having an open line of communication between the two of you is imperative. If you decide against getting a personal trainer, you may still want to have someone on your team to confide in about this new lifestyle change.

When it comes to weight and the public stigma behind it, we often fear exposing ourselves and becoming vulnerable to others.

A personal trainer can be a middle ground for this concern. They are your sounding board, but also your source of information during the process. They might not always say what you want them to, but they are there to guide you, not be your friend.

After all, it's best that they know as much as possible and you are learning tools to help you along the way!

Here are a few ways to open up to your personal trainer.

Establish A Rapport: Get to know each other. Ask about their credentials, tell them about yourself, and just be friendly. Make sure your personal trainer is open to casual dialogue and isn't just telling you how to do squats or lifts.

Be Honest: Are you someone who likes to smear cake frosting on graham crackers? You're probably not alone. You should feel comfortable telling your personal trainer without fear of judgement. They will help you beat that habit.

Swap Shoes: Not physically, but mentally. If you're meeting with a trainer because you gained weight after a nasty divorce, then tell exactly what happened. Then, picture yourself as the personal trainer with a client just like you. This will help you understand each other, and therefore get the most out of your personal training sessions.

Tip #5: Mix Things Up

Forgive the pun, but variety really is the spice of life. If all you do when you work out is run on the treadmill, then eventually you will get bored, and so will your body. This happens even if you love to run!

It's also important to work each muscle group differently, otherwise things may grow stagnant and your weight loss will plateau. Our muscles like variety, too!

Every trainer should make sure that their client stays engaged and interested in their workout. While there is nothing wrong with repetition; the truth is that a workout should remain stimulating in the sense that you are working on the different parts of your body.

Make sure that you are switching things up from time to time, whether it's focusing on a different set of muscle groups each day, or trying out new cardio routines or stretching exercises. Or perhaps even a different environment!

Here are a few tips to help you mix things up.

Different Body Parts: Exercise a different body part each day. For example, do an ab workout Monday and Friday, and legs Tuesday and Thursday. You will find that isolating specific groups will help thoroughly work out those specific groups!

Schedule Rest Days: Not only does your body need a day off, but so does your mind. Make sure to schedule one or two rest days a week. While you should refrain from doing intense activity on those days, it's still a good idea to stretch.

Look into some basic stretching techniques or consider taking yoga!

Tip #6: Healthy Eating

It is important to eat a well-balanced diet in order to get the most out of your workouts. One supports the other and without a healthy eating plan in place, your fitness routines will only help to sustain your current weight, not help you slim down.

Your doctor, and your personal trainer decide on what foods you should and shouldn't be eating, then you can move forward in your healthy lifestyle, taking the tools given beyond the walls of the gym.

Here are a few tips to remember when it comes to nutrition and the body.

Never Skip a Meal. You may think that skipping breakfast will help you with your goal, but that's far from the truth. Personal trainers will often help to remind you of the importance of eating food at every meal. If this is something you do all the time, make sure to let them know beforehand. Let's face it though, just because you eat, doesn't mean it's healthy. Make sure to always eat foods that fit within your lifestyle change.

Food Is Fuel: Personal trainers will help you understand, that just like cars need gasoline, human bodies need food. This is especially important to remember if you have ever had an unhealthy relationship with food.

Even though you'd never put bad gas in your car, you still need to put gas in it. The same goes with food and our bodies. You want to remember to put the healthiest and most nutrient rich foods on your plate in order to nourish your body, not just feed it.

Factor in Small Snacks: Our stomachs are like our fuel tanks. If they get empty, we can't go very far. Just think about the times between meals when your stomach announces its presence. It's sort of like the gas light coming on in our cars! This can be the most vulnerable time in our day, and the time we are at the most risk of grabbing something fast and unhealthy. So, make sure you plan small, healthy snacks in between meals.

Tip #7: Replace Old Habits

Grocery shopping, for some of us, has become almost robotic, a task done out of necessity, tucked neatly into our lives. But has your quick and precise grocery shopping routine become outdated? If you are throwing cartons of ice cream and bags of chip in the cart, it's definitely time to regroup.

Unfortunately for most of us, old habits die hard. Which is why your personal trainer is going to select a slow and steady pace from the beginning.

Here are a few helpful tips on how to begin changing those old habits.

Swap Out One Food Each Week. If you go from buying nothing but frozen pizzas and ice cream, to loading up your cart with chicken, veggies and whole grains, it won't be long before your body starts to crave junk food. Swap out one bad food with one healthy one each week when you shop. For example, replace a regular carton of ice cream with a low-fat version of your favorite flavor!

Don't Give Up When It's Hard. If you are still in a physical condition that dictates an inability to complete a workout without pausing for rest, that's okay.

Instead of ending your workout right then and there, pause, take a couple of minutes to catch your breath, stretch, and regroup, and pick up exactly where you left off.

You will notice as time passes that you will be able to make it through your workouts without that pause.

Stop Hitting the Snooze Button. If you're looking to become healthier and stronger, then you should embrace taking care of your body. This includes resting your body for as long as it needs.

Commit to going to bed at a decent time and getting up as soon as that alarm goes off. Pretend as though your alarm clock doesn't even have a snooze button!

Setup Everything the Night Before: Our mornings are often rushed as we're trying to get ready, which means that we may not exercise or take the time to eat right. Make it a habit to get everything ready for the next day, before you go to bed.

Layout your clothes, setup your coffee maker, pack your lunch, etc. Do as much as possible beforehand, and you will notice just how much time you have to spare, and how motivated you are to stay healthy!

Tip #8: Choosing Supplements

With so many supplements on the market, it can be a bit nerve-racking trying to find the right one for you. Those who are looking to lose weight and lower their cholesterol have different needs than someone who wants to gain weight or muscle.

After discussing your goals with your personal trainer, they may suggest adding supplements to your diet. For example, someone who needs to lose weight because of obesity but hates eating fish would benefit from odorless fish oil supplements.

Are you looking to add muscle mass to your physique? A personal trainer may want you to add creatine to your diet, which is a supplement that provides you with more energy during your power lift sessions.

Other supplements that a personal trainer may recommend include daily multivitamins, calcium, probiotics, and vitamin c. If your doctor says that you have high blood sugar, your personal trainer may suggest a supplement that helps prevent the absorption of excess blood sugar.

As mentioned in a previous chapter, it is vital that you communicate all health issues with your personal trainer from the beginning. Supplements are not replacements for the nutrients your body needs, but can help you replenish your sources.

Tip #9: Beyond Weight Loss

Having a personal trainer on your side is not only positive because of the motivation and knowledge they bring, but as a constant reminder that exercise and healthy eating are not just about weight loss. It's about becoming the best version of yourself. It's looking to a longer, leaner and heathier future.

A healthy lifestyle will strengthen your muscles, your lungs, your heart, your posture, your bones, and your overall physique. But a healthy and balanced routine will also improve your mental acuity. Doctors will oftentimes prescribe exercise and healthy eating to help treat diseases such as Anxiety, Depression, and ADHD.

A good personal trainer will always recognize the importance of a healthy mind and strong body when introducing you to a new lifestyle. Without a strong mind, changing your lifestyle could be nearly impossible. Exercise and healthy eating are truly an all-encompassing affair, feeding you from the inside out.

Make sure to discuss with your personal trainer the non-physical issues you may suffer from. Your personal trainer will be able to tailor your workout and your eating around who you are as an individual and oftentimes this knowledge is imperative to your success.

Tip #10: Rest & Recover

When you first begin to consider hiring a personal trainer, beyond the excitement of a newer and better you, your mind may begin to throw out those dreaded subtractions you think you'll have to make to your life. You will think about the ice cream, pizza, wine, beer, and lazy 6 hour naps every Sunday.

Each one of the above things bring you pleasure in some way. Usually, they produce endorphins in your brain, the chemical that makes you happy. But just because you are taking those out, doesn't mean you won't be adding in healthy lifestyle choices that will give you the same gleeful feeling.

For everything you're giving up, there's something to be gained.

Here are some things your personal trainer may add to your lifestyle.

Delicious New Recipes: Not all healthy food involves flavorless kale and boiled chicken. It doesn't matter how healthy something is, most people won't eat it if its bland or off-putting. But thanks to the internet, you now have access to thousands-if not millions-of recipes that are good for you and delicious!

And who knows, maybe you'll actually love the taste of kale!

New Activities: Yes, many of us would much rather

lounge around in our sweats than bust a sweat on an exercise machine. But your personal trainer will remind you on the daily that there's so much more to exercise than just boring machines.

Many gyms offer exercise classes like aerobics, yoga, cycling, and-if you're up for a challenge-CrossFit! Not to mention the other things you can do as exercise outside of the gym. Hiking, biking, swimming, rock climbing, and running are just a few.

Meeting New People: It takes commitment to go to the gym when we would much rather be at home, but you're bound to meet new people the more often you go.

No matter what stage of fitness and health someone is in, they are still there for the same general reason as you, to be the best version of them they can be.

Often, finding a support system from these people can help to keep you on track and accountable.

Conclusion

If you want to get in the best shape of your life, there will be real sacrifices that you will have to make. You'll need to be consistent about fitness and make it a real priority. You will also have to take the time to make sure that you are adequately celebrating your wins while holding yourself accountable.

You might also have to remain conscious about your relationships. It can be very challenging to get fit if you have a close friend or significant other who tries to tempt you into unhealthy activities, or has anything negative to say about your journey. It's up to you to make sure that you let these people know that you are serious about your fitness journey.

Ultimately, your body and mind will thank you for getting fit. The road might not always be easy, but you can do this!

Resources

Here is a link to a resource that I believe will help you:

Tips from Personal Trainers:
>>https://www.afpafitness.com/blog/personal-training-tips-for-your-clients

The American Fitness Professionals Association (AFPA) is an organization that educates individuals on being the healthiest version of themselves that they can be.

Thank you for purchasing my book as I hope I have in some way helped you in your journey to a healthier you.

Troy Esprit

Troy Esprit

www.pro7fitness.com